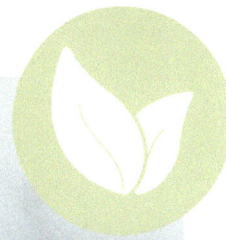

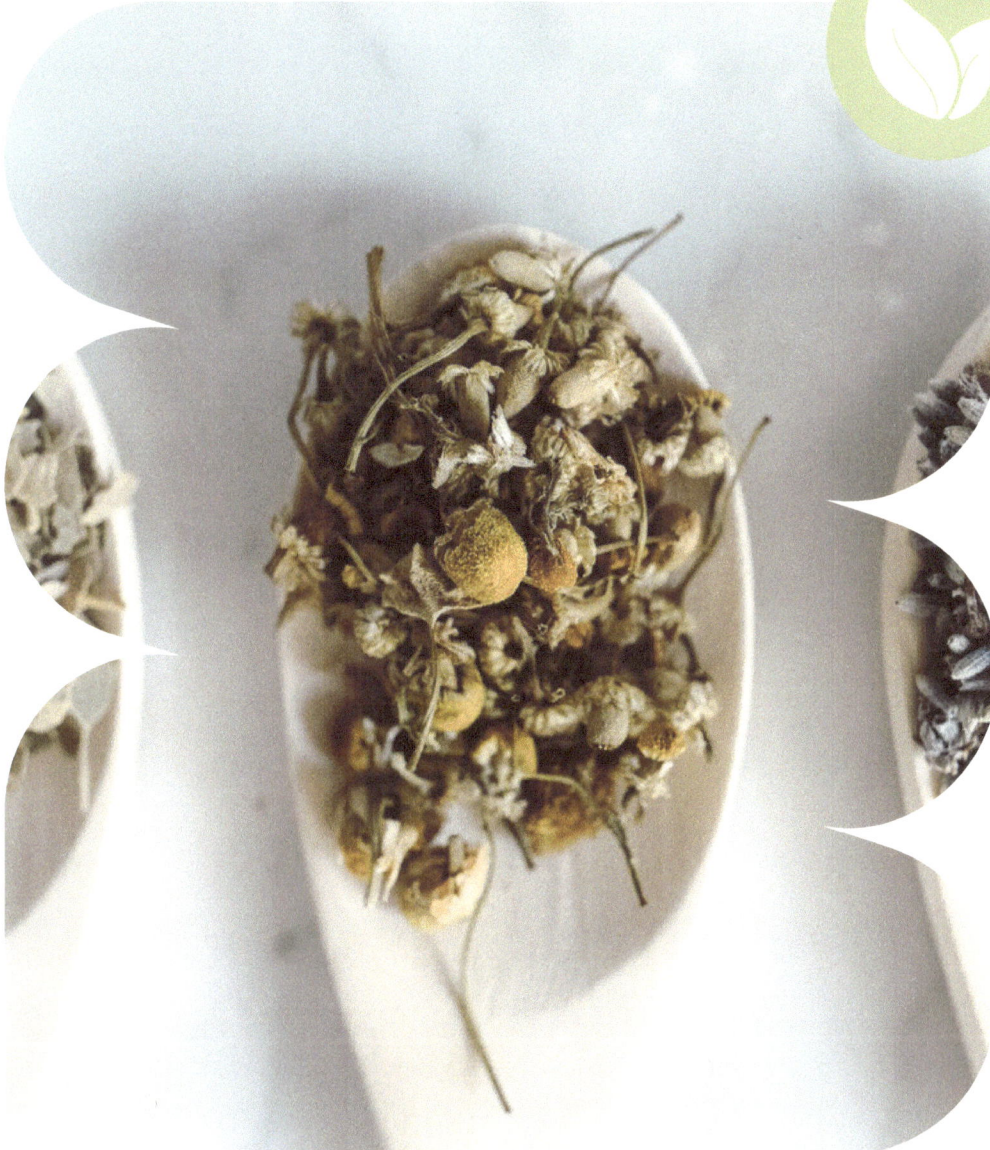

# HERBAL REMEDIES FOR DETOXIFICATION

*The ABCs of Clean Living*

BY ASHLEY REYES

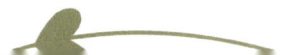

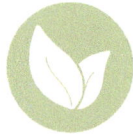

## TABLE OF CONTENTS

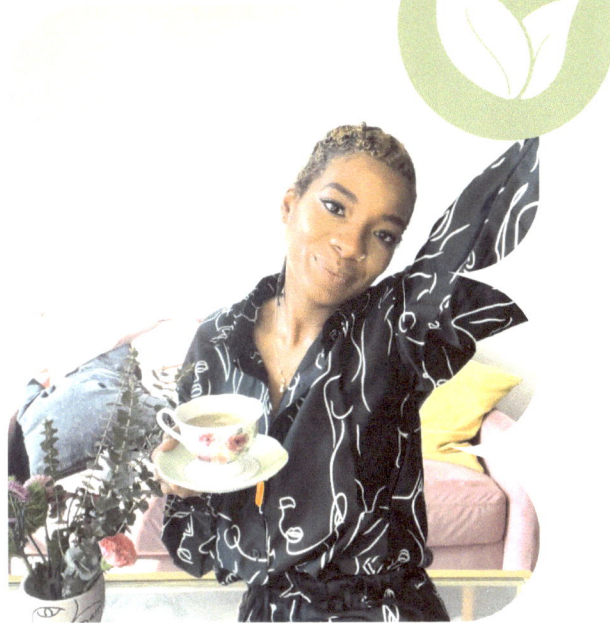

Once a month, without fail, my mother would prepare a special breakfast feast for us: fluffy pancakes, crispy turkey bacon, and perfectly scrambled eggs. It was always a treat, and my siblings and I eagerly looked forward to it. But the highlight, or so we thought, was the glass of juice that accompanied the meal. Little did we know, that juice held a secret ingredient.

Every time, without exception, my mother managed to trick us with that juice. It wasn't just any ordinary juice; it was juice with a generous dose of castor oil. The moment we took a sip, we'd realize what she had done, but by then, it was too late. I used to think it was her way of getting back at me for all the mischief I'd caused that month. It felt like her subtle revenge for every broken vase, every spilled drink, and every sibling argument.

But as I grew older, I began to see the truth behind this ritual. My mother wasn't punishing us; she was caring for us in the most loving way she knew. Adding castor oil to our juice was her method of detoxifying our bodies, flushing out the toxins that accumulated over time. It was a tradition rooted in her desire to keep us healthy and strong.

This was my first introduction to the concept of herbal detoxes and their incredible benefits. My mother's monthly concoction was more than just a mischievous trick; it was a lesson in the importance of cleansing and nurturing our bodies. That simple act of mixing castor oil with juice planted the seeds of my fascination with herbalism and natural health.

Today, as I practice herbalism, I often think back to those mornings. What once seemed like a dreaded part of breakfast has become a cherished memory and a cornerstone of my journey into the world of herbal detoxification. My mother's loving care and wisdom continue to inspire me, reminding me of the powerful connection between nature and health.

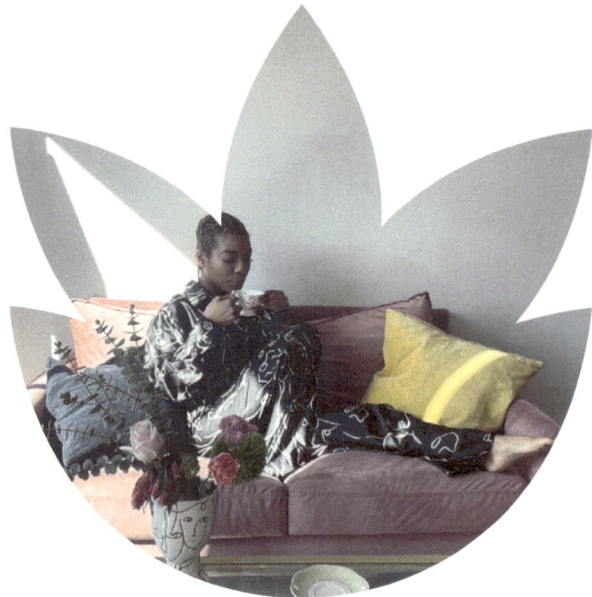

# INTRODUCTION

Welcome to *Herbal Remedies for Detoxification: The ABCs of Clean Living*, your vibrant companion on the journey to a toxin-free life.

This ebook is designed to guide you through the process of detoxifying your body using natural, herbal remedies. In today's fast-paced world, our bodies are exposed to numerous toxins from the environment, food, and lifestyle choices. Detoxification is essential to maintaining optimal health and well-being.

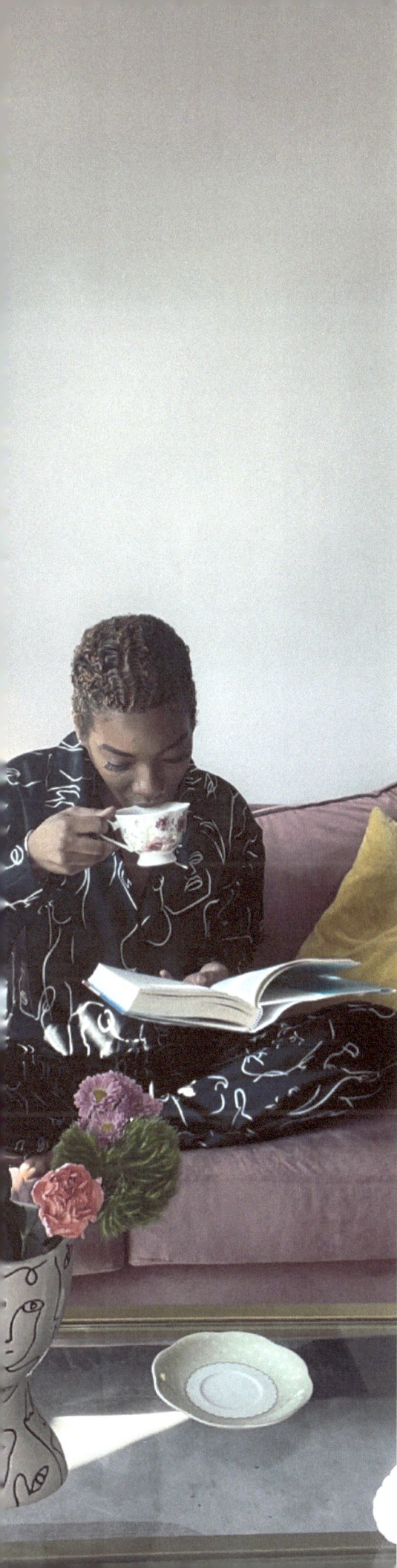

# Understanding Detoxification

Detoxification is the process of removing toxins from the body. It involves cleansing the blood, liver, kidneys, and other organs to improve overall health. Toxins can come from various sources such as pollutants, chemicals, processed foods, and stress.

The human body has its own natural detoxification systems, primarily carried out by liver, kidneys, intestines, lungs, lymphatic system, and skin. These systems work together to process and eliminate toxins that accumulate from various sources.

# The Importance of Detoxification

While the body is equipped to handle a certain level of toxins, modern life often introduces more than it can efficiently manage. Over time, the accumulation of toxins can lead to various issues, including:

- Chronic fatigue
- Digestive problems
- Skin issues
- Allergies and sensitivities
- Mental fog and lack of clarity
- Weight gain and metabolic issues
- Weakened immune system

Detoxification helps to alleviate these issues by supporting and enhancing the body's natural processes, allowing it to function more efficiently and effectively.

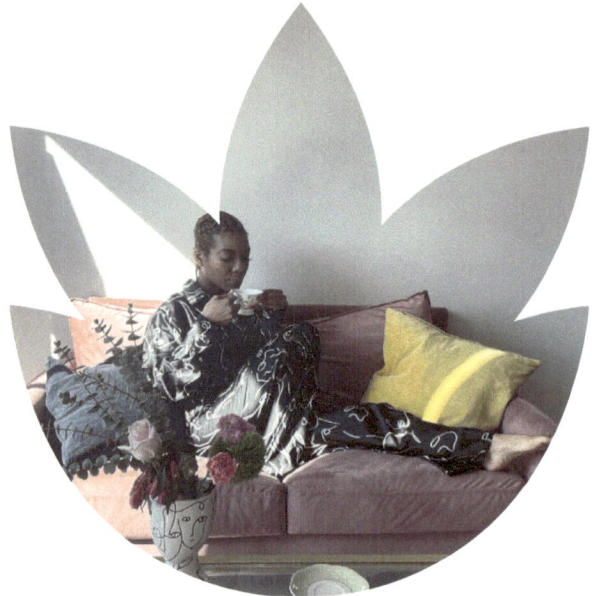

# HISTORY OF HERBALISM DETOXIFICATION

Herbalism is one of the oldest medical practices, extending back thousands of years. Herbs were employed for healing and purification by ancient civilizations including the Egyptians, Chinese, and Native Americans. Detoxification, as part of traditional medicine, has its roots in Ayurveda and Traditional Chinese Medicine, with an emphasis on balance and impurity removal. In this eBook, "Herbal Remedies for Detoxification: The ABCs of Clean Living," we'll look at how these ancient traditions might be incorporated into modern life to promote better health and wellness.

# The Ancient Art of Herbalism

Herbalism has a long history, dating back to ancient civilizations that recognized the natural connection between nature and health.

## Egyptians

One of the earliest groups of people to record the usage of herbs for therapeutic purposes was the Egyptians. They used herbs with medicinal and purifying powers, such as garlic, coriander, and mint. Garlic, for example, was prized for its blood cleansing and immunity-boosting properties. These techniques were extensively recorded on papyrus scrolls, demonstrating the Egyptians' advanced mastery of herbal therapy.

## Chinese

Focusing on preserving equilibrium inside the body, Traditional Chinese Medicine (TCM) is an all-encompassing method that has been used for thousands of years. Because of their ability to promote health and aid in detoxification, herbs like ginger, ginseng, and licorice root are essential in Traditional Chinese Medicine. For example, ginseng is utilized to increase energy and stress tolerance, and licorice root balances the effects of other herbs and aids in body detoxification.

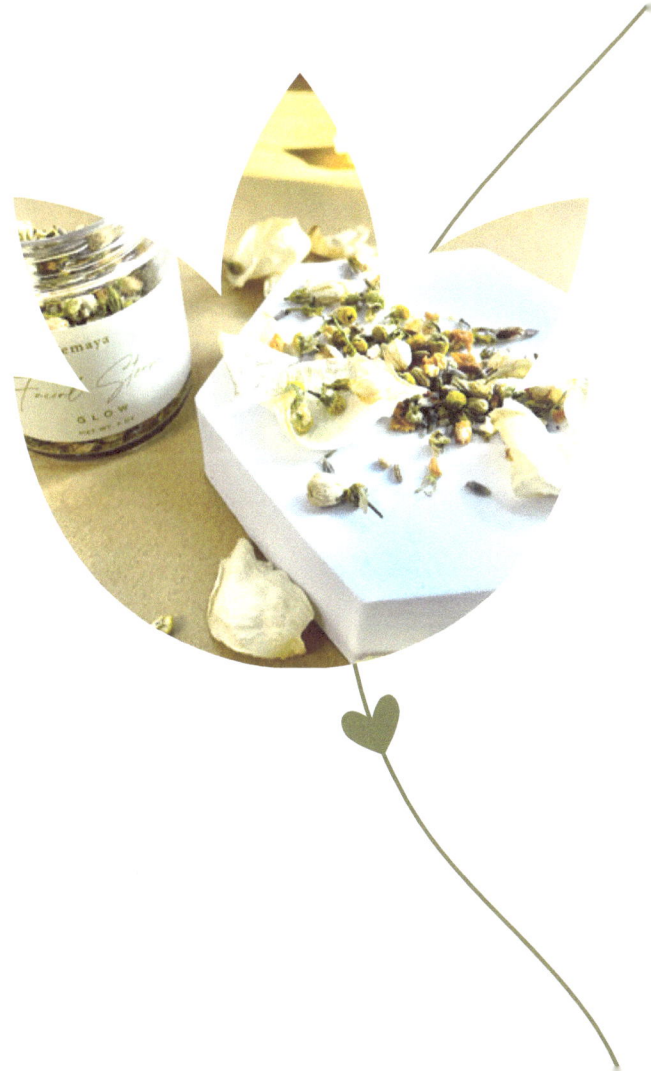

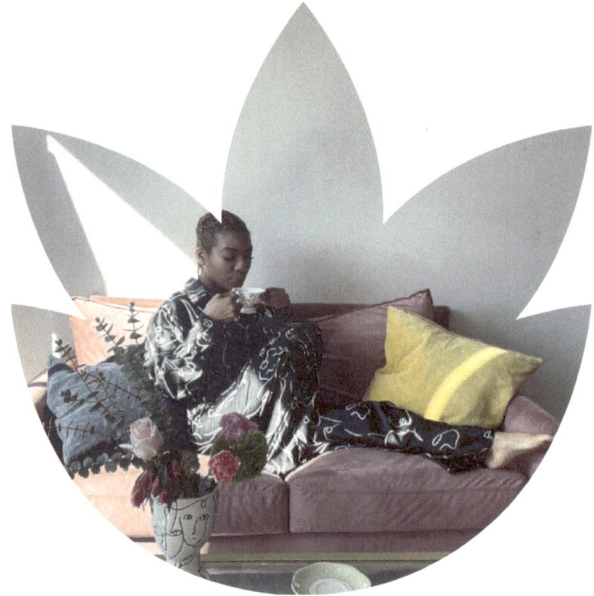

# BENEFITS OF DETOXIFICATION

# IMPROVED DIGESTION

Cleansing the digestive system enhances nutrient absorption.

Digestion is the foundation of health, influencing how our bodies absorb nutrients and eliminate waste. Poor digestion can cause a variety of problems, including bloating, constipation, and nutritional deficits. Herbal cleansing can help improve digestive health in a variety of ways.

Dandelion root, ginger, and fennel are said to help cleanse the digestive tract by increasing the production of digestive enzymes and bile. This aids in the more effective breakdown of food and reduces waste accumulation.

Garlic and oregano are natural antimicrobials that can help balance the gut microbiome. Proper digestion and nutrition absorption require a healthy gut flora.

# INCREASED ENERGY

Fatigue and low energy levels are frequent concerns in today's society. Herbal detoxification can naturally raise energy levels by eliminating toxins that weigh the body down and assisting the body's natural energy generation mechanisms.

Toxins can disrupt cellular energy production, an essential process that occurs within our cells' mitochondria. Mitochondria, recognized as the cell's powerhouses, alter nutrients into adenosine triphosphate (ATP), the cell's primary energy currency. Toxins can affect mitochondrial activity, resulting in less ATP generation and, as a result, lower energy levels.

Milk thistle has been shown in several trials to have liver-protective results. The main ingredient in milk thistle, silymarin, contains antioxidant and anti-inflammatory properties that help to protect liver cells from toxic damage. Milk thistle helps with detoxification by improving liver function, helping the liver to eliminate toxic compounds more effectively from the bloodstream. This decrease in toxin levels can ease the stress on the mitochondria, resulting in increased cellular energy generation.

# BETTER SKIN HEALTH

The skin is the body's largest organ and serves as a mirror of our overall health. Toxins, bad food, and lifestyle choices can all cause skin disorders such as acne, eczema, and premature aging. Herbal detoxification can revitalize the skin from the inside out by cleaning the body and supplying necessary nutrients.

Toxins in the body can lead to a variety of skin issues. Certain herbs may aid in the detoxification process, helping to eliminate harmful poisons and resulting in better skin. Herbs such as burdock root and neem have long been used to purify the blood, thereby removing toxins that might cause skin problems.

The root of the burdock plant was used to heal skin sores by Native American tribes such as the Menominee and Micmac, as well as a range of diseases by the Cherokee. It was also supposed to aid in the elimination of toxins from the bloodstream, potentially reducing the prevalence of skin conditions such as acne and eczema.

04

# ENHANCED MENTAL HEALTH

Mental clarity and emotional well-being are important aspects of total health. Herbal detoxification can significantly improve mental health by lowering the weight of pollutants that impair brain function and mood. The accumulation of toxins in the body can adversely affect brain function and mood, leading to issues such as brain fog, anxiety, and depression. Herbal detoxification can have a profound impact on mental health by reducing the burden of toxins and supporting the body's natural detoxification processes.

Stress is a common factor that can exacerbate the effects of toxins on mental health. Adaptogenic herbs help the body adapt to stress and balance cortisol levels, which are often elevated in response to stress.

Cognitive function can be significantly impaired by the presence of toxins in the body. Herbs that improve blood circulation to the brain and support detoxification processes can enhance memory, focus, and overall cognitive performance.

# STRONGER IMMUNITY

A strong immune system is vital for protecting the body from infections and illnesses. Toxins can impair immunological function, increasing susceptibility to sickness. Herbal detoxification can boost the immune system by assisting with the elimination of toxic toxins while also supplying nutrients that promote immunological health.

Antioxidants serve an important function in protecting the body from oxidative stress, which may compromise its immune system. Herbal detoxification is the intake of antioxidant-rich herbs that neutralize free radicals and promote general immunological health.

Green tea contains catechins, which are potent antioxidants. These substances assist to protect cells from free radical damage, reduce oxidative stress, and boost immunological function. Regular use of green tea can boost the body's ability to fight infections and preserve overall health.

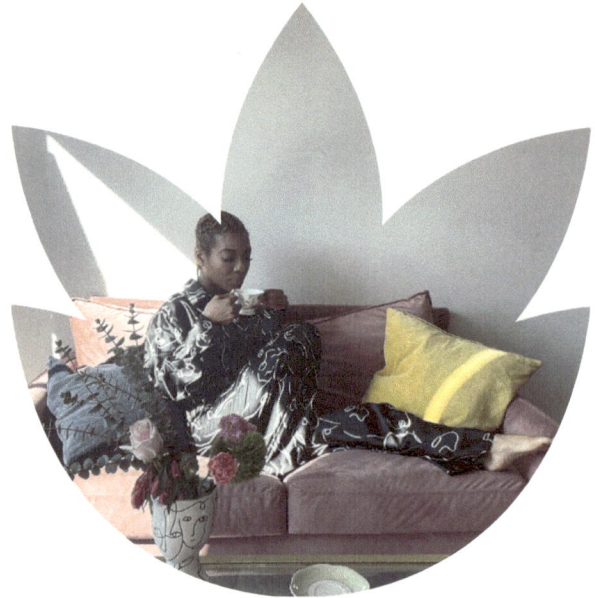

# THE ABC'S OF HERBAL DETOXIFICATION

# A - ASTRAGALUS

Often used in traditional Chinese medicine, astragalus boosts the immune system and supports liver function, aiding in the detoxification process.

Therapeutic Actions:
Adaptogen
Anti-Hypertensive
Immunomodulator
Tonic

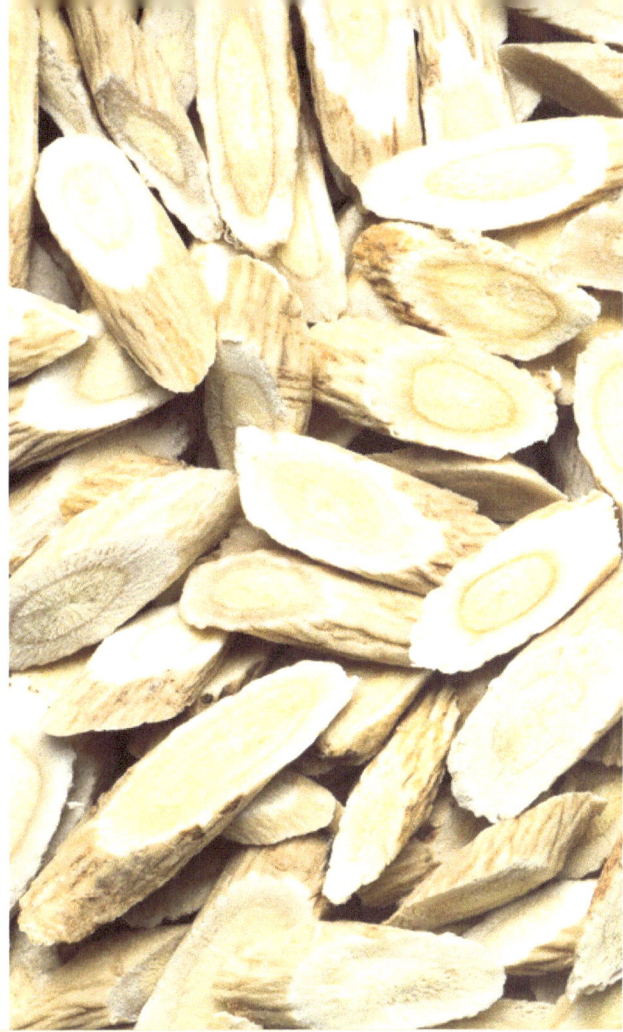

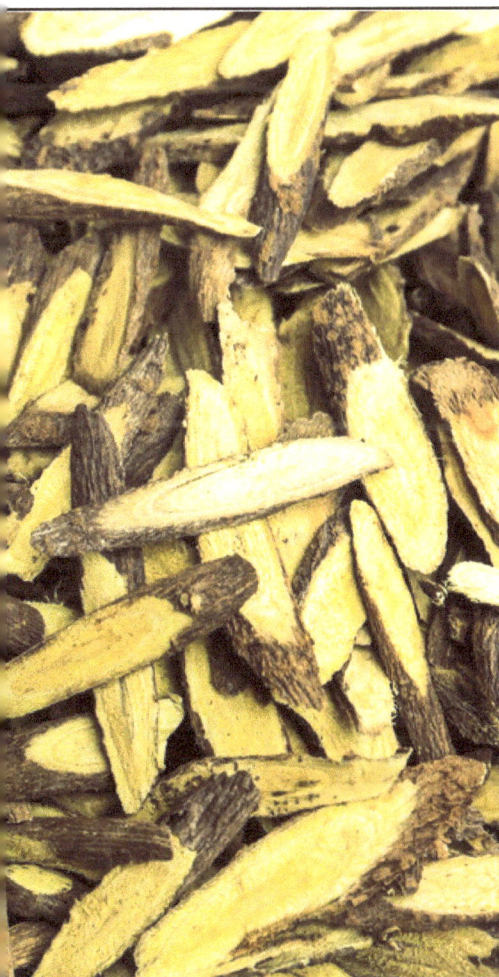

# B - BURDOCK ROOT

Burdock root is a powerful blood purifier and supports liver detoxification. It helps in removing heavy metals and other toxins from the blood

Therapeutic Actions:
Antioxidant
Anti-Inflammatory
Diuretic

# C - CILANTRO

Cilantro is effective in binding to heavy metals and helping to remove them from the body. It's often used in heavy metal detox protocols.

Therapeutic Actions:
Anti-Bacterial
Anti-Inflammatory
Diuretic
Stimulant

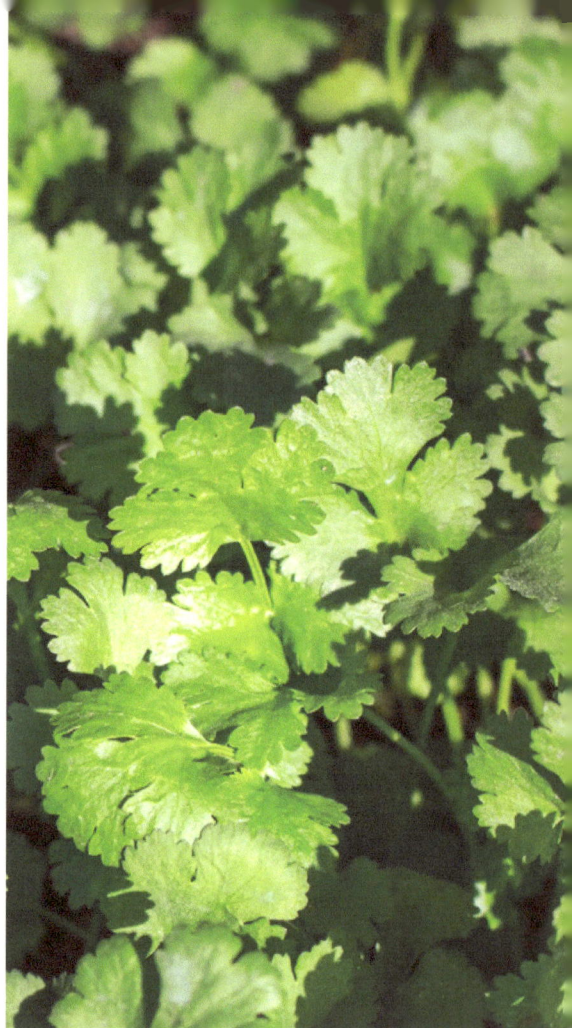

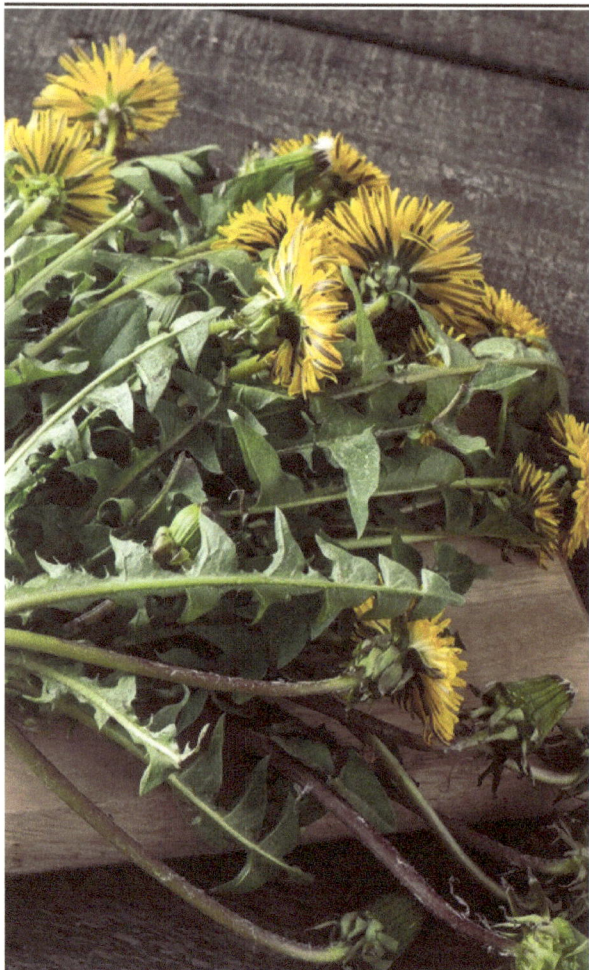

# D - DANDELION

Dandelion is a potent liver cleanser and diuretic, helping to flush toxins from the body. It also supports kidney function.

Therapeutic Actions:
Alterative
Bitter
Cholague
Diuretic
Hepatic

# E - ECHINACEA

Echinacea strengthens the defenses against illness and strengthens the immune system. Additionally, it aids in lymphatic cleansing.

Therapeutic Actions:
Anti-Catarrhal
Anti-Microbial
Immunostimulant

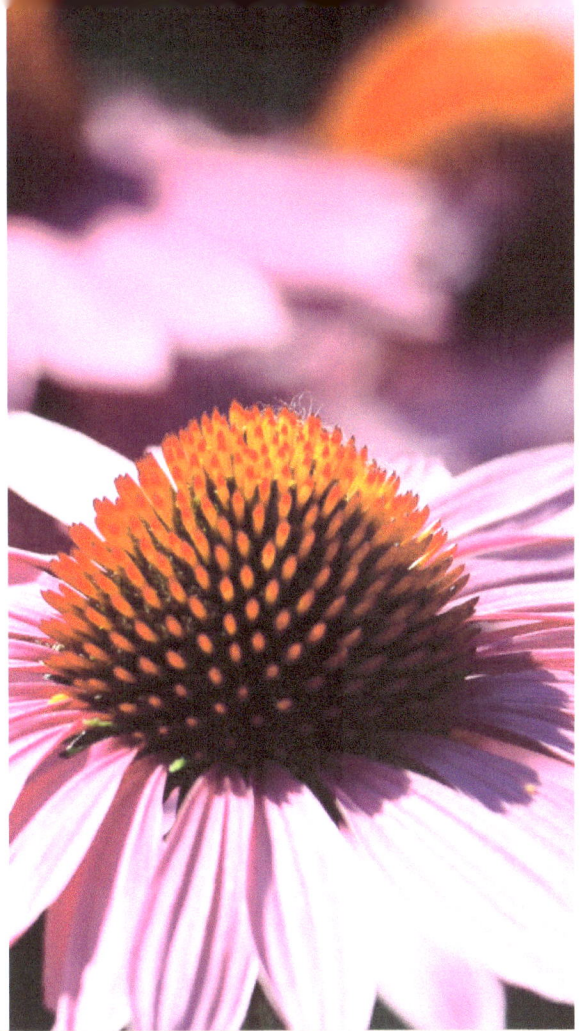

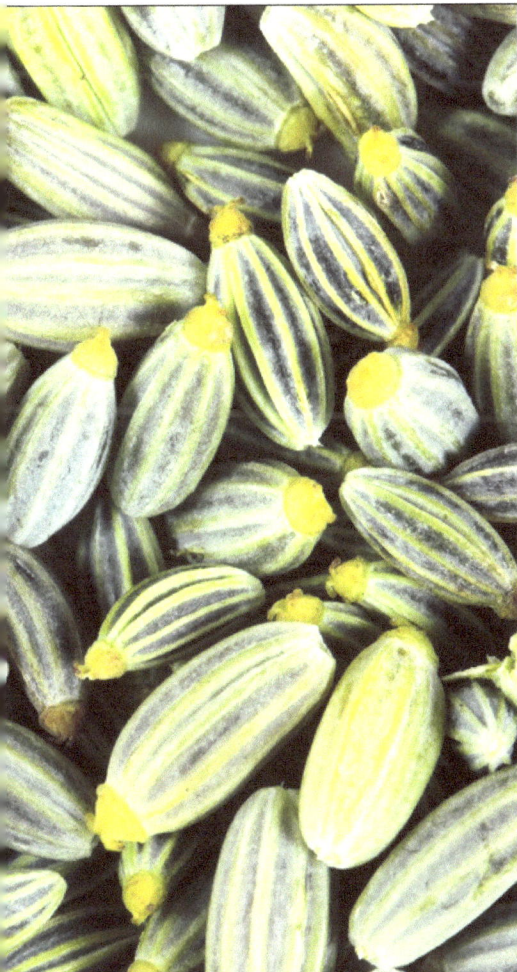

# F - FENNEL

Fennel is excellent for digestive detoxification, reducing bloating and cleansing the digestive track.

Therapeutic Actions:
Anti-Spasmodic (Respiratory System)
Carminative

# G - GREEN TEA

Green tea is rick in antioxidants and supports liver detoxification. It also boosts metabolism and aids in weight loss.

Therapeutic Actions:
Vaginal Health Weight Management

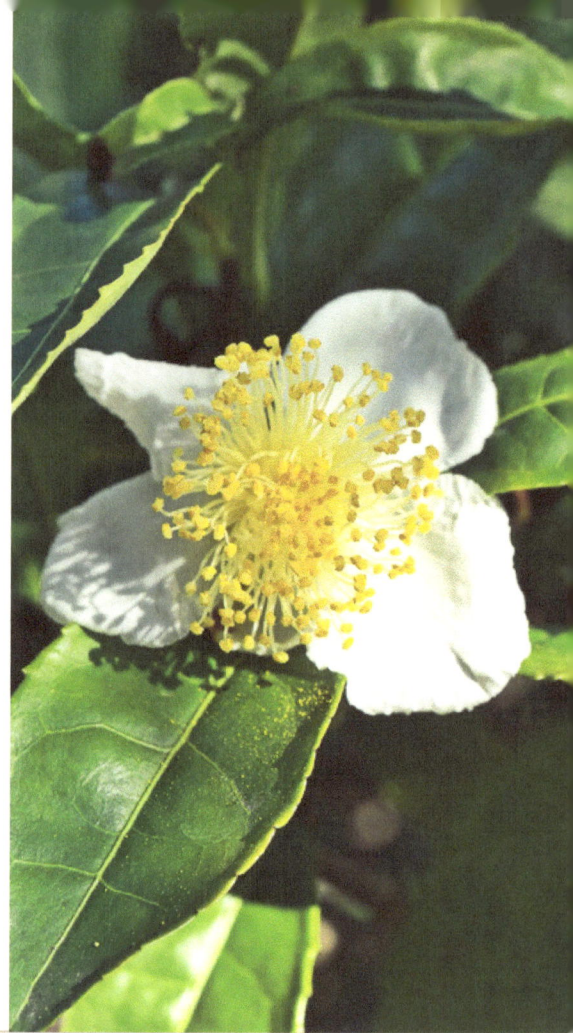

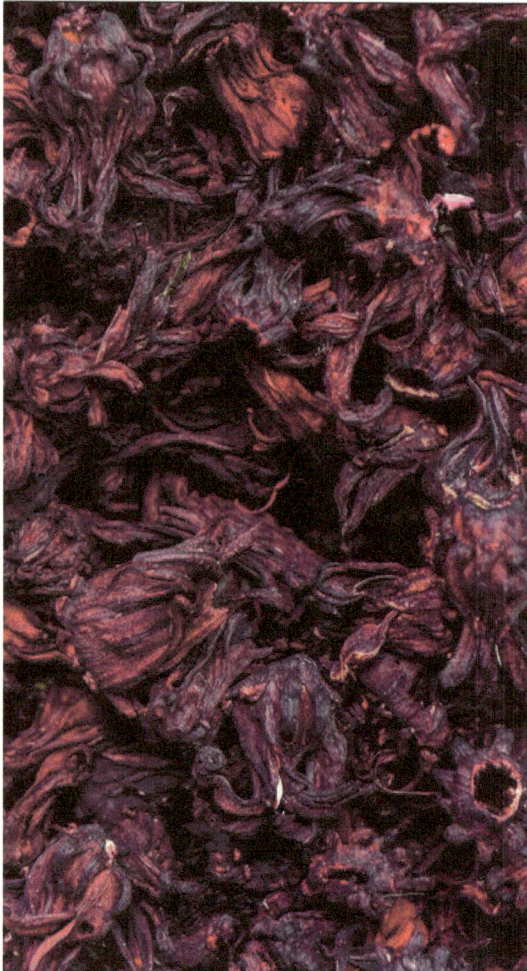

# H - HIBISCUS

Hibiscus tea is a gentle diuretic and helps in flushing toxins through increased urination. It also supports liver health.

Therapeutic Actions:
Anti-Inflammatory
Diuretic Laxative

# I - INDIAN GOOSEBERRY (AMLA)

Amla is a powerful antioxidant and supports liver detoxification. It is also beneficial for skin health.

Therapeutic Actions:
Anti-Parasitic
Diuretic
Immunomodulator
Promote Hair Growth

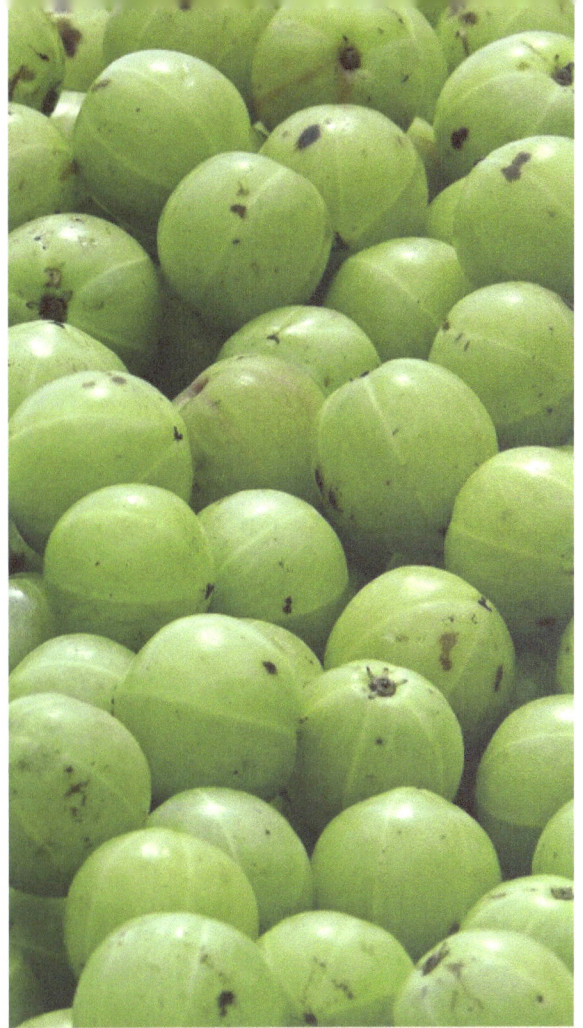

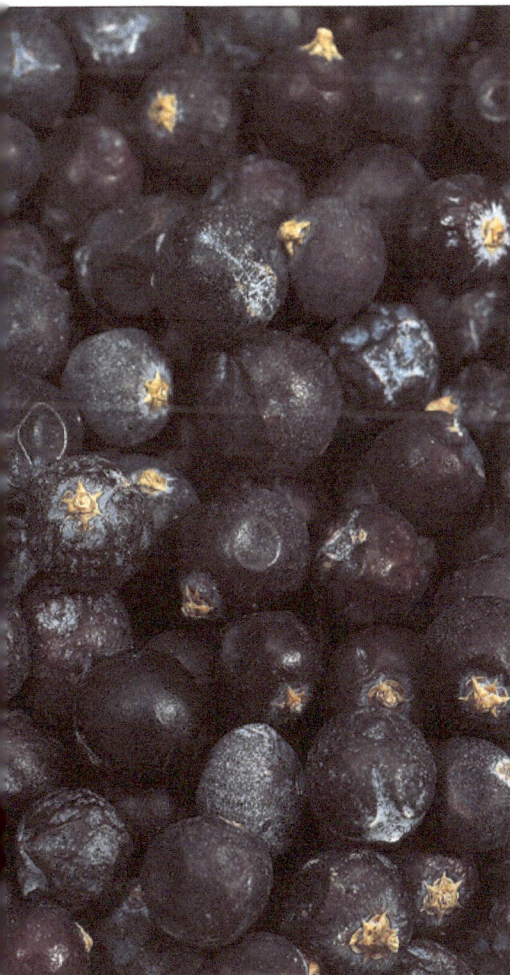

# J - JUNIPER BERRY

As a natural diuretic, juniper berry aids in kidney and urinary tract detoxification.

Therapeutic Actions:
Anti-Rheumatic
Anti-Septic Diuretic
Emmagogue

# K - KUDZU

Kudzu is helpful in substance addiction detox regimens because of its reputation for hepatotoxic properties and its capacity to reduce alcohol cravings.

Therapeutic Actions:
Antioxidant
Anti-Inflammatory
Estrogen Balancing
Immune Stimulator

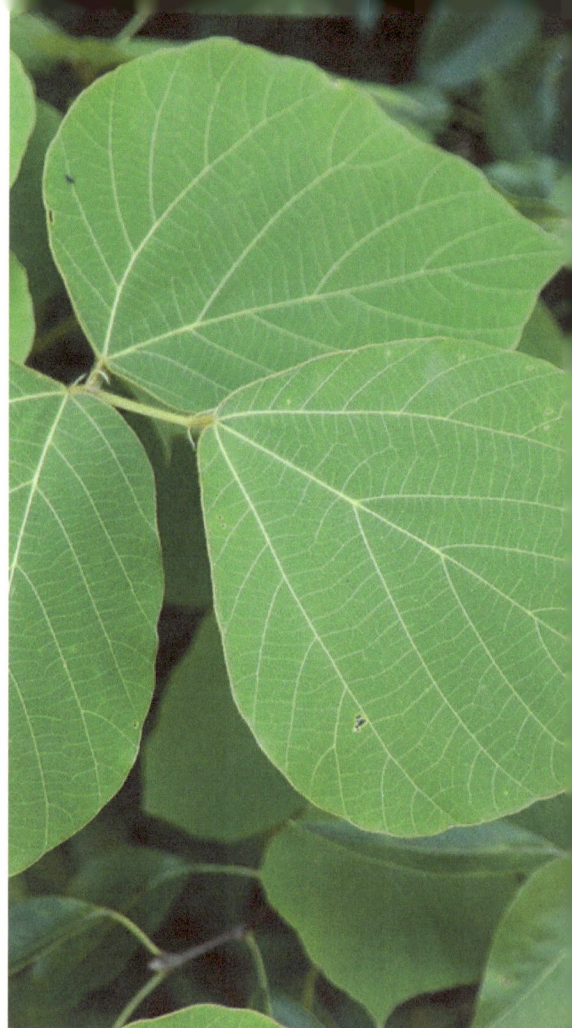

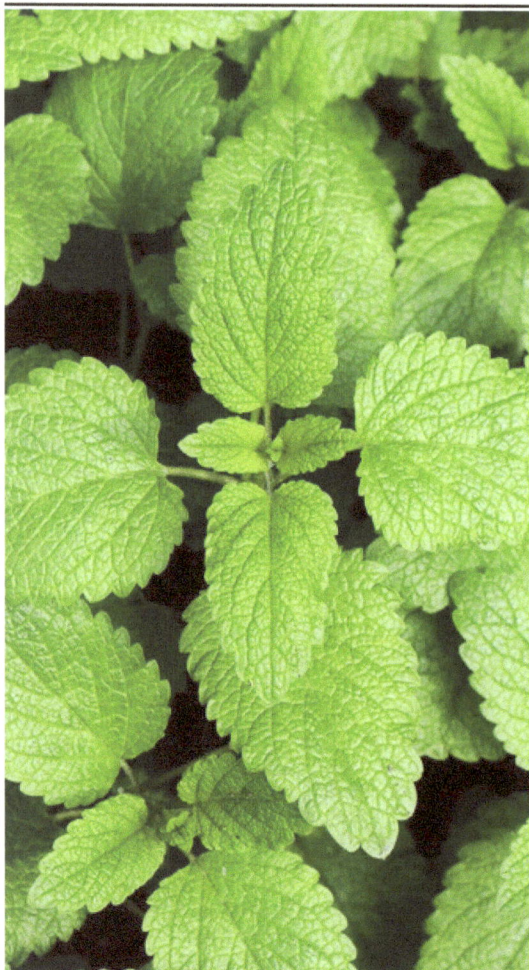

# L - LEMON BALM

Lemon balm calms the nervous system and promotes the functioning of the liver and digestive system.

Therapeutic Actions:
Anti-Inflammatory (Nervous)
Anti-Microbial
Nervine (Cardiovascular System)

# M - MILK THISTLE

One of the most well-known liver detoxifiers is milk thistle, which shields and regenerates liver cells.

Therapeutic Actions:
Hepatic
Mucilaginous
Nutritive

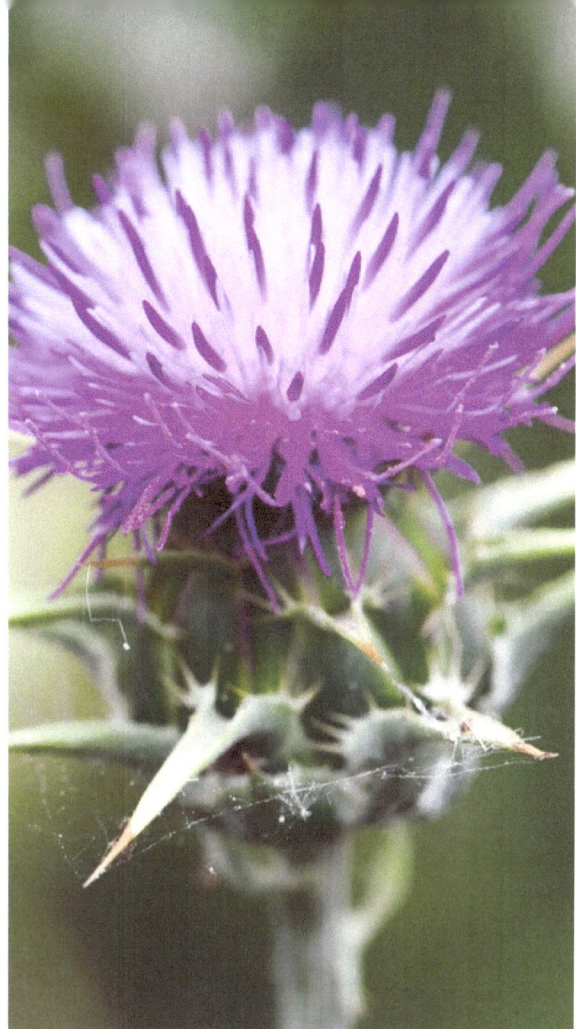

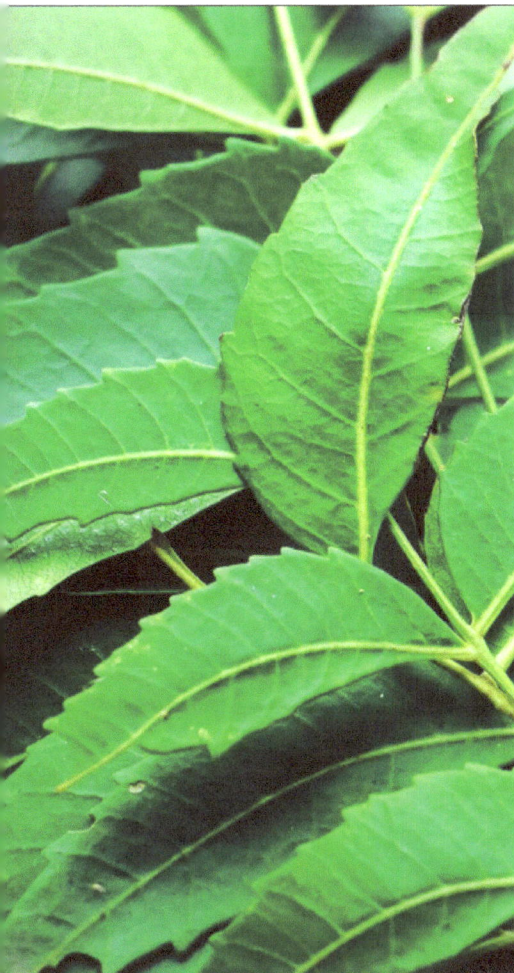

# N - NEEM

Neem promotes healthy skin and is an effective blood purifier. Because of its antimicrobial qualities, it is frequently employed in detoxification regimens.

Therapeutic Actions:
Anti-Bacterial
Antioxidant
Antipyretic

# O - OREGANO

With potent antibacterial qualities, oregano aids in cleansing and promotes healthy digestion.

Therapeutic Actions:
Anti-Bacterial
Anti-Microbial
Anti-Viral
Bronchodilator

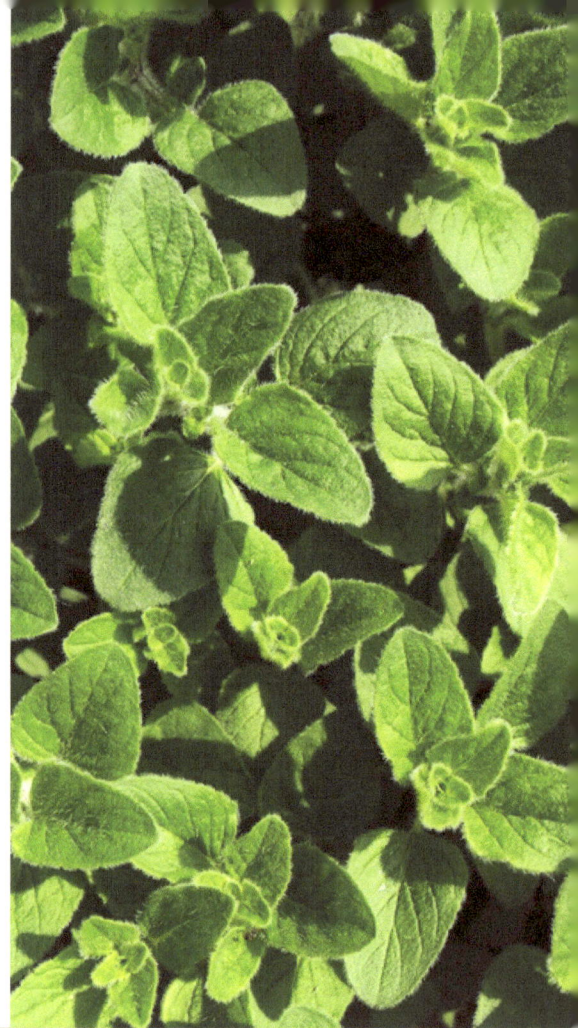

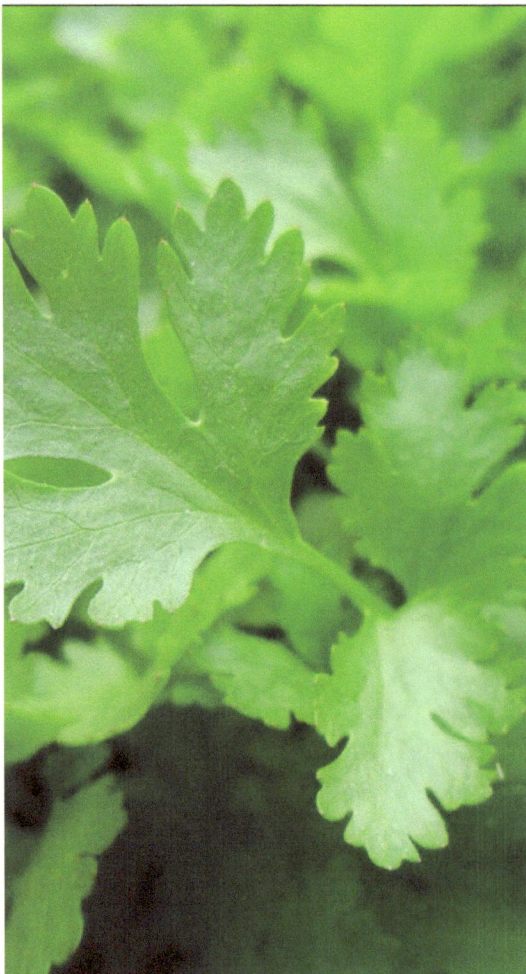

# P - PARSLEY

Parsley aids in kidney cleansing and acts as a natural diuretic. Furthermore, it has a lot of minerals and vitamins.

Therapeutic Actions:
Anti-Septic
Carminative
Diuretic
Hypotensive
Parasiticide

# Q - QUASSIA

Because it gets rid of parasites and has cleansing qualities, quassia is used to enhance digestive health.

Therapeutic Actions:
Anti-Bacterial
Anti-Fungal
Anti-Parasitic

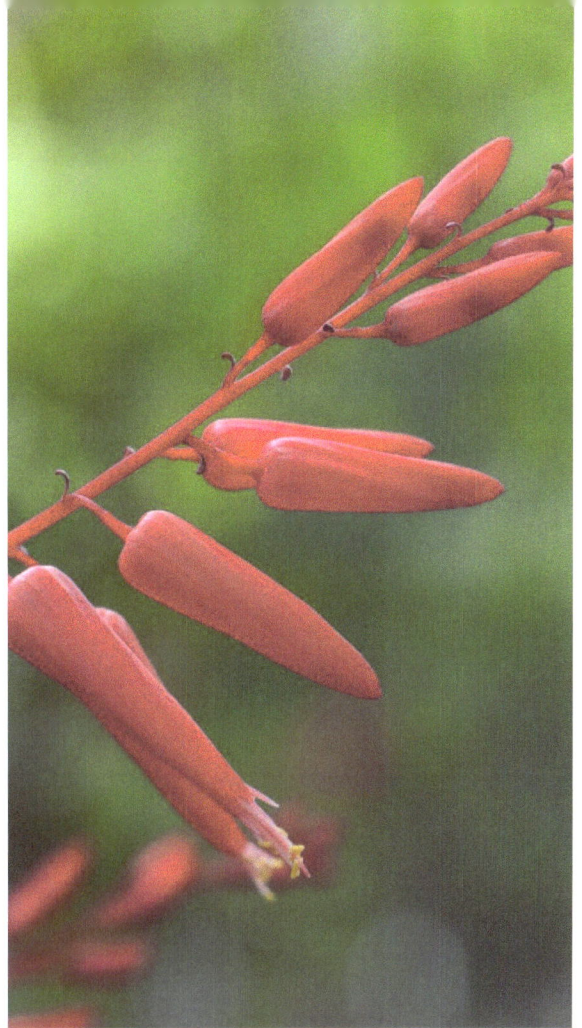

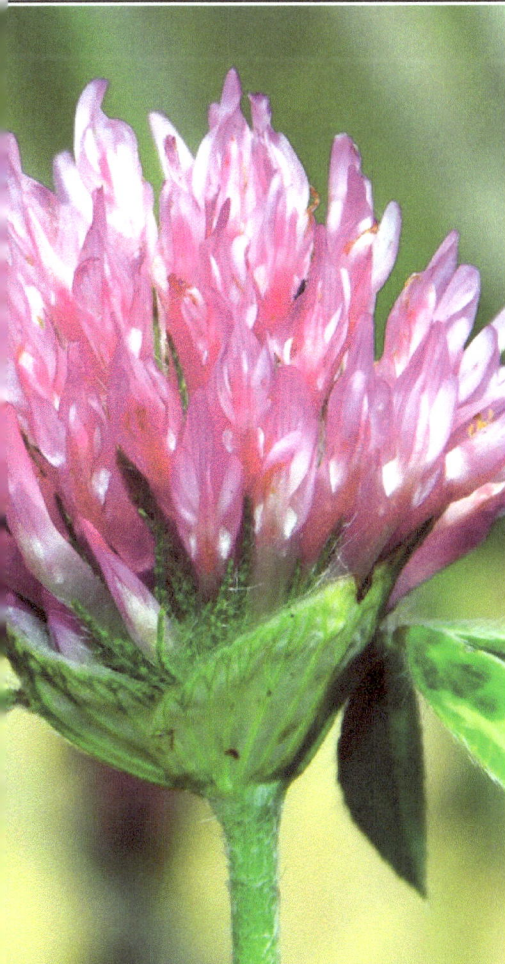

# R - RED CLOVER

Red clover aids in lymphatic cleansing and is a blood purifier. It also supports healthy skin.

Therapeutic Actions
Alterative
Anti-Spasmodic
Diuretic
Expectorant

# S - SPIRULINA

Rich in antioxidants and chlorophyll, spirulina is a superfood that promotes general cleansing.

Therapeutic Actions:
Nutritive
Tonic

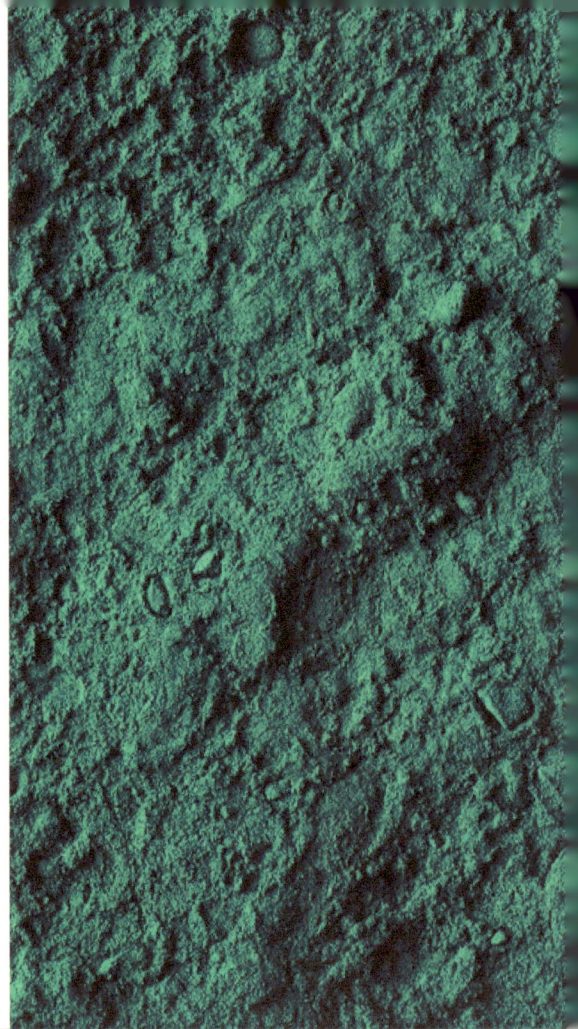

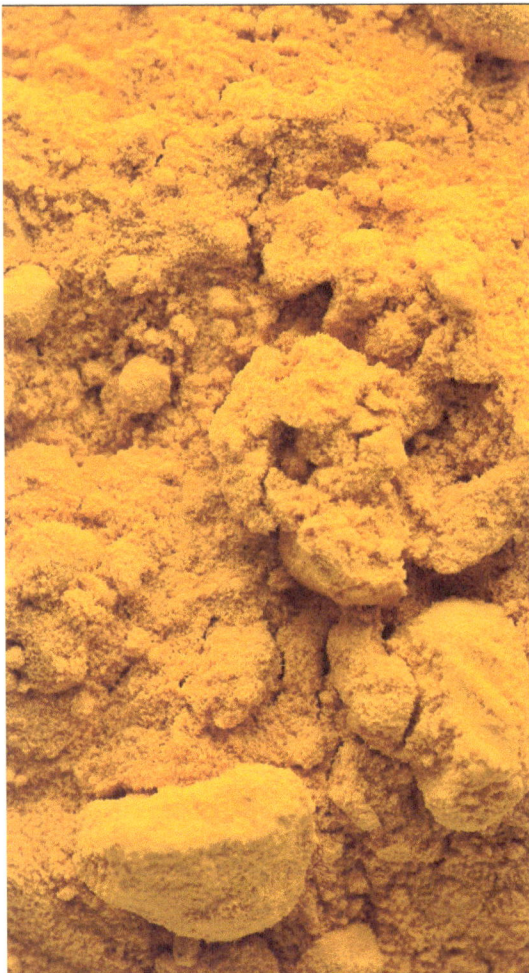

# T - TURMERIC

Turmeric has potent anti-inflammatory properties and aids in liver detoxification. It facilitates digestion as well.

Therapeutic Actions:
Aromatic
Anti-Inflammatory
Astringent
Cardio-Protective

# U - UVA URSI

Uva Ursi promotes kidney function and is useful in cleansing the urine tract.

Therapeutic Actions:
Anti-Catarrhal
Anti-Lithic
Astringent
Bitter Diuretic

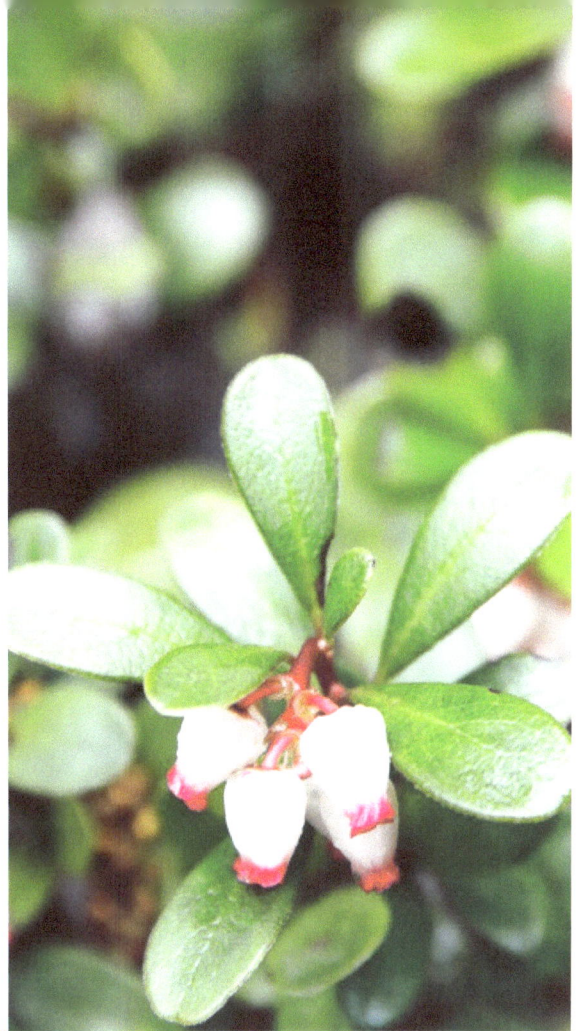

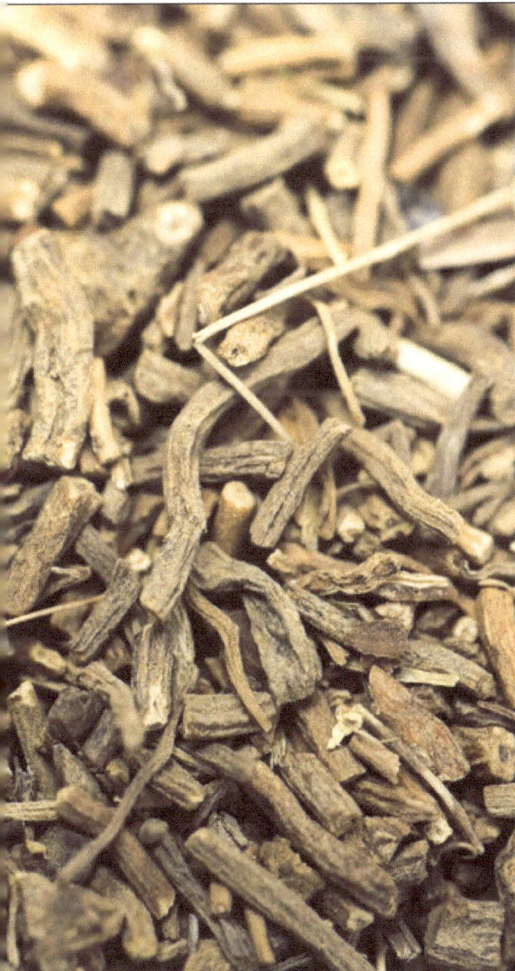

# V - VALERIAN ROOT

Valerian Root promotes nervous system health and detoxifies the body of stress-related toxins.

Therapeutic Actions:
Anti-Spasmodic
Carminative
Hypnotic
Hypotensive
Nervine

# W - WHEATGRASS

Wheatgrass is very alkalizing and aids in overall detoxification. It's high in vitamins, minerals, and chlorophyll.

Therapeutic Actions:
Blood Cleanser
Blood Builder
Blood Purifier
Nutritive
Tonic

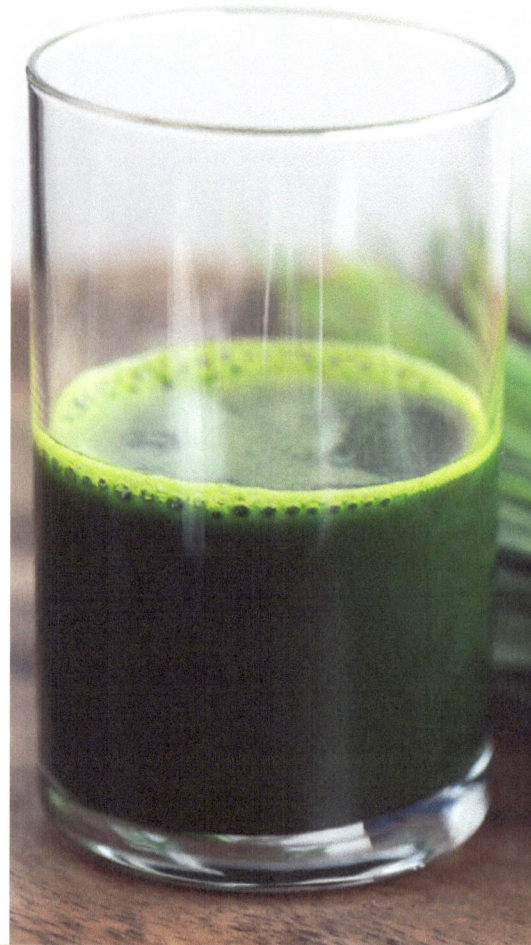

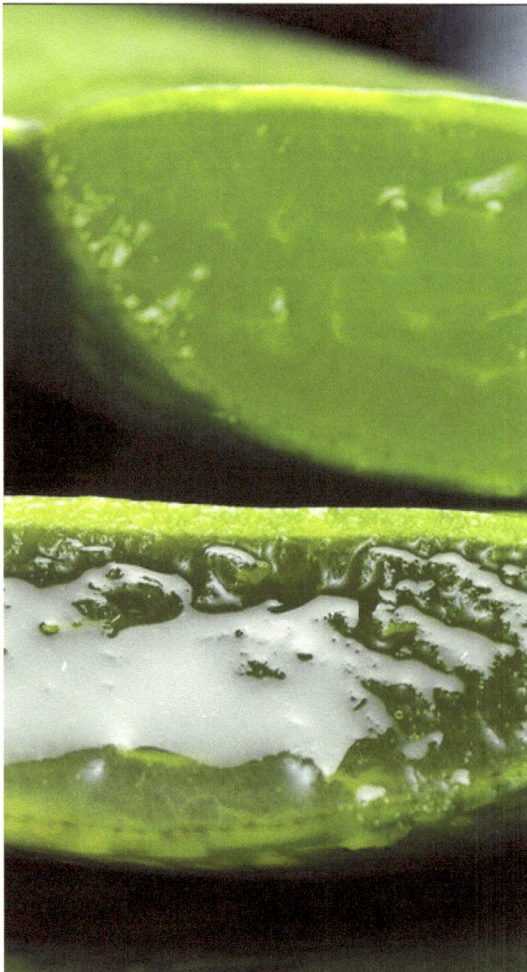

# X - XEROPHYTE (ALOE VERA)

Aloe Vera, a xerophyte, is effective for skin and intestinal detoxification.

Therapeutic Actions:
Anti-Septic
Emmenagogue
Hemostatic
Purgative
Tonic

# Y - YARROW

Yarrow promotes liver and intestinal cleansing while also benefiting skin health.

Therapeutic Actions:
Anti-Inflammatory
Astringent
Carminative
Hemostatic
Tonic

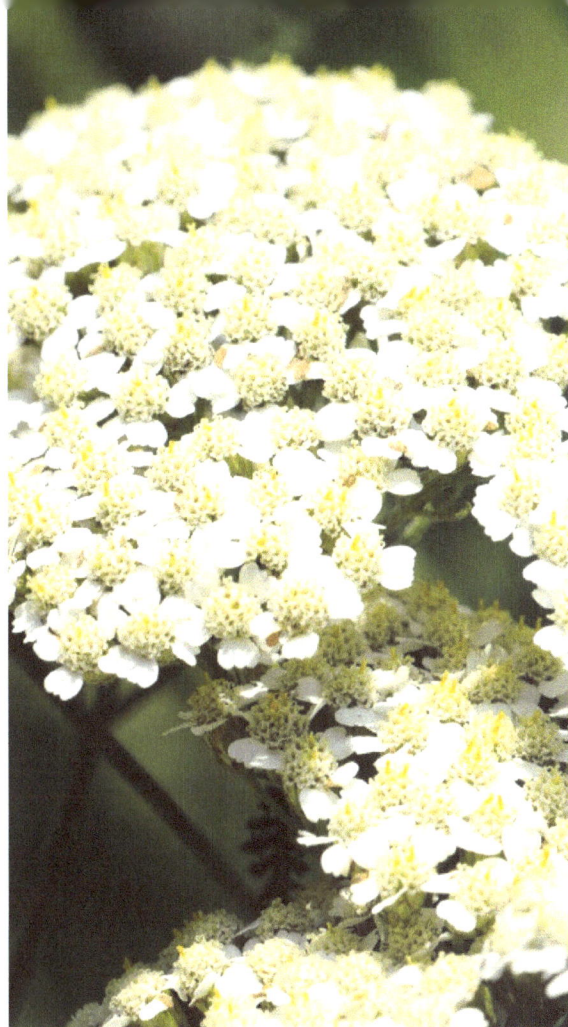

# Z - ZEOLITE

Zeolite is a mineral that assists the body in detoxifying heavy metals and other pollutants.

Therapeutic Actions:
Antioxidant
Anti-Microbial
Anti-Viral
Detoxification

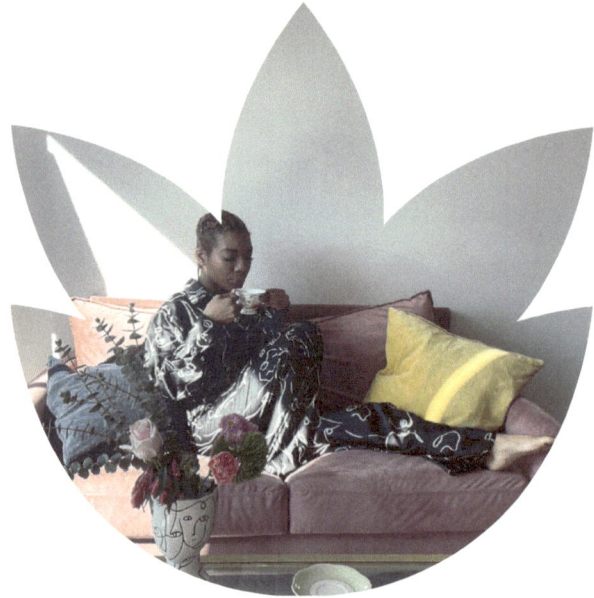

# HERBAL DETOX RECIPES

# LIVER DETOX TEA

**Dandelion and Milk Thistle Tea**

Ingredients:

- 1 tablespoon dried dandelion root
- 1 teaspoon crushed milk thistle seeds
- 1 teaspoon dried peppermint leaves (optional for flavor)
- 1 tablespoon honey (optional)
- 2 cups water

Instructions:

1. Bring the water to a boil in a saucepan.
2. Add the dandelion root and milk thistle seeds to the boiling water.
3. Reduce the heat and let it simmer for 10-15 minutes.
4. Add peppermint leaves if desire, and let steep for another 5 minutes.
5. Strain the tea into a cup.
6. Add honey to taste.
7. Stir well and enjoy.

# LIVER DETOX TEA

**Turmeric and Ginger Tea**

Ingredients:

- 1 teaspoon turmeric powder ( or 1-inch fresh turmeric root, sliced)
- 1-inch fresh ginger root, sliced
- 1 tablespoon honey (optional)
- 1 lemon, juiced
- 2 cups water

Instructions:

1. Bring the water to a boil in a saucepan.
2. Add the turmeric and ginger to the boiling water.
3. Reduce the heat and let it simmer for 10-15 minutes.
4. Strain the tea into a cup.
5. Add honey and lemon to taste.
6. Stir well and enjoy.

# KIDNEY DETOX TEA

**Nettle and Parsley Tea**

Ingredients:

- 1 tablespoon dried nettle leaves
- 1 tablespoon dried parsley leaves
- 1 tablespoon honey (optional)
- 2 cups water

Instructions:
1. Bring the water to a boil in a saucepan.
2. Add the nettle and parsley leaves to the boiling water.
3. Reduce the heat and let it simmer for 10 minutes.
4. Strain the tea into a cup.
5. Add honey to taste.
6. Stir well and enjoy.

# KIDNEY DETOX TEA

**Cornsilk and Horsetail Tea**

Ingredients:

- 1 tablespoon dried corn silk
- 1 tablespoon dried horsetail
- 1 tablespoon honey (optional)
- 2 cups water

Instructions:

1. Bring the water to a boil in a saucepan.
2. Add the corn silk and horsetail to the boiling water.
3. Reduce the heat and let it simmer for 10 minutes.
4. Strain the tea into a cup.
5. Add honey to taste.
6. Stir well and enjoy.

# BRAIN FOG DETOX TEA

**Ginkgo Biloba and Rosemary Tea**

Ingredients:

- 1 tablespoon dried ginkgo biloba leaves
- 1 teaspoon dried rosemary leaves
- 1 tablespoon honey (optional)
- 2 cups water

Instructions:

1. Bring the water to a boil in a saucepan.
2. Add the ginkgo biloba and rosemary leaves to the boiling water.
3. Reduce the heat and let it simmer for 10 minutes.
4. Strain the tea into a cup.
5. Add honey to taste.
6. Stir well and enjoy.

# BRAIN FOG DETOX TEA

**Lemon Balm and Peppermint Tea**

Ingredients:

- 1 tablespoon dried lemon balm leaves
- 1 tablespoon dried peppermint leaves 1
- tablespoon honey (optional) 2 cups
- water

Instructions:
1. Bring the water to a boil in a saucepan.
2. Add the lemon balm and peppermint leaves to the boiling water.
3. Reduce the heat and let it simmer for 10 minutes.
4. Strain the tea into a cup.
5. Add honey to taste.
6. Stir well and enjoy.

PRACTICING MINDFULNESS AND MEDITATING DAILY CAN HELP YOU UNLOCK INNER PEACE AND DETOX THE MIND.

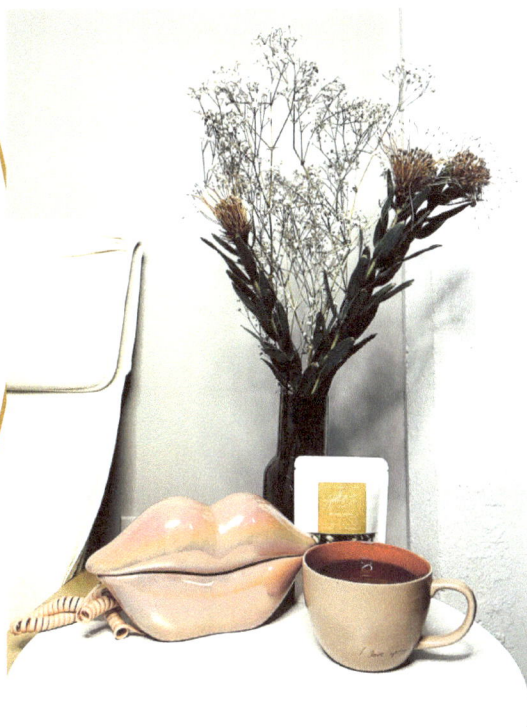

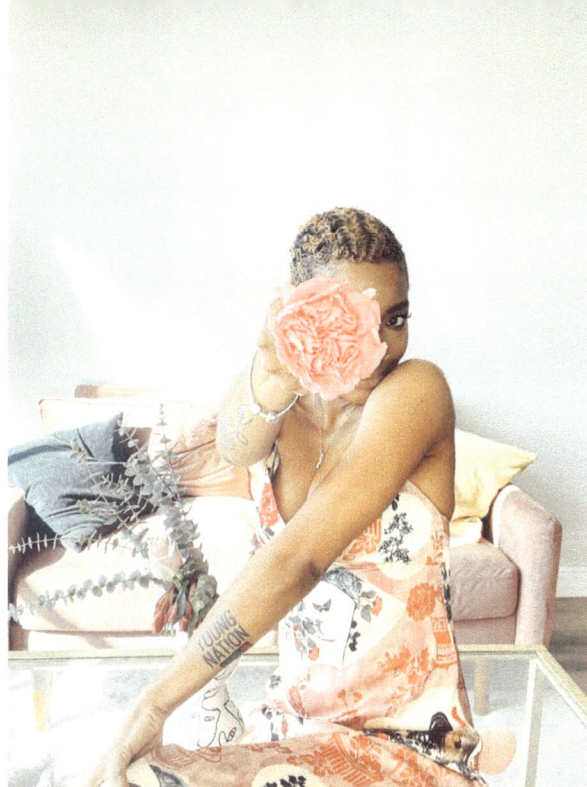

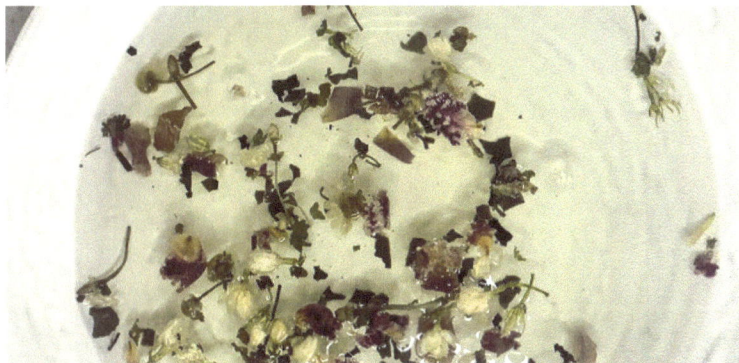

These herbal teas are intended to aid in the cleansing and proper functioning of the liver, kidneys, and brain. You may effectively assist your body in getting rid of toxins, lowering inflammation, and improving your general health by including these natural remedies into your daily routine. Drinking these teas on a regular basis maymay strengthen immunity, increase energy, and improve cognitive function. These herbal mixes provide a safe and efficient means to enhance health and energy, regardless of your goals—improving your liver's capacity to purify your blood, aiding your kidneys in eliminating waste, or improving your mental acuity. Incorporate them into your overall health regimen to support an active lifestyle and a well- balanced diet.

Do not drink if you are pregnant or may be pregnant. As a reminder, consult with your doctors before using these recipes as an aid to any and all illnesses.

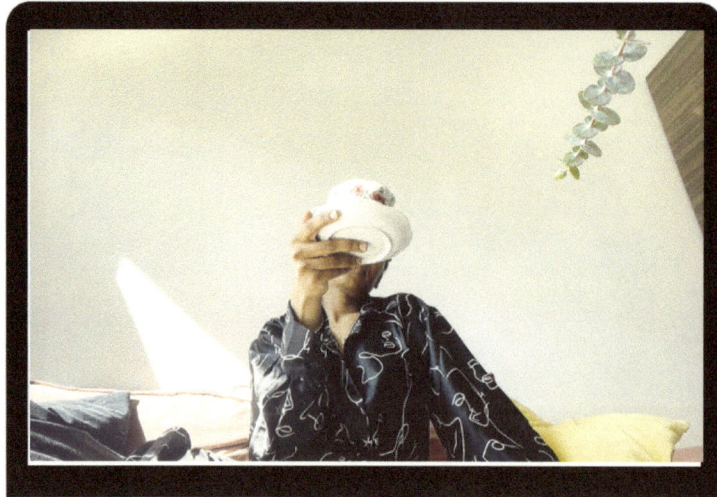

Yemaya is a tea and herbal company created to provide you with everything you need for divine femininity.

#areyoufeelingdivine

# REFERENCES

Balch, P. A. (2006). Prescription for Herbal Healing. Avery Publishing Group.

Bone, K., & Mills, S. (2013). Principles and Practice of Phytotherapy: Modern Herbal Medicine. Churchill Livingstone.

Dave. (2023, May 17). Burdock. Achula.https://www.achula.com/post/burdock

Dharmananda, S. (2002). The Use of Herbs in Chinese Medicine. Institute for Traditional Medicine.

Foster, S., & Hobbs, C. (2002). The Peterson Field Guide to Western Medicinal Plants and Herbs. Houghton Mifflin Harcourt.

Gladstar, R. (2012). Rosemary Gladstar's Medicinal Herbs: A Beginner's Guide. Storey Publishing.

Murray, M. T., & Pizzorno, J. (2005). The Encyclopedia of Healing Foods. Atria Books.

ND, J. R. (2015). The Little Herb Encyclopedia, 4th Edition. Woodland Publishing.

Nunn, J. F. (2002). Ancient Egyptian Medicine. University of Oklahoma Press.

Ulbricht, C., Basch, E., Basch, S., Bent, S., Boon, H., Burke, D., ... & Wagner, J. (2008). Echinacea (Echinacea angustifolia, E. pallida, E. purpurea): Systematic Review by the Natural Standard Research Collaboration. Journal of Dietary Supplements, 5(2), 94-124.

Winston, D., & Maimes, S. (2007). Adaptogens: Herbs for Strength, Stamina, and Stress Relief. Healing Arts Press.

Zhang, T. (2009). Traditional Chinese Medicine Approaches to Detoxification and Internal Cleansing. Chinese Journal of Integrative Medicine.

Milton Keynes UK
Ingram Content Group UK Ltd.
UKHW050222021224
451567UK00009B/77